Ketogenic Diet

for Rapid Weight Loss:

Recipes and Mistakes to Avoid

By

Michelle Brighton

Table of Contents

Introduction

Unless you have been living under a rock somewhere, you have probably heard about ketogenic diets – where the aim is to restrict your carb intake to such a point that your body is actually forced to switch over from using glucose as its primary energy source to using fat.

Maybe you read about it online or heard about it from a friend and are curious to see whether or not this diet can actually work for you. If you are anything like me, you are no doubt skeptical that this is just another fad diet that gives unsustainable results. In fact, when I first read about the ketogenic diet, I was convinced that it sounded a little too good to be true – you get to lose weight, feel fantastic and you never even get hungry? No diet I had ever tried before had been able to give me more energy and I was generally starving at the end of the day.

Now, that was fine when my motivation levels were high at the outset but, as time went by, motivation would flag and I would give in. Not only would I not maintain any weight loss, but I was losing the fight overall – I would end up heavier than when I started. And it was not from a lack of discipline or trying either – you name a diet and I will no doubt have tried it in the past – to this day, I still cannot face the idea of eating cabbage and I cringe at the sight of lettuce.

When I started researching the ketogenic diet, I had pretty much given up. I was going to give it a good old college try but, in all honesty, I did not expect to see real results. (I think I really just wanted to be able to justify drinking fresh cream.) So I gave it a go and, during the first week, I felt terrible. (I am not going to lie – switching your body's main fuel source is tough at first.)

I lost six pounds in the first week alone and that motivated me to keep going.

The switch for me seemed to happen almost overnight – I went from feeling like I was coming down with the flu to being full of energy and raring to go. I could concentrate better and think more clearly. But, best of all, I was not hungry at all.

I went from coming home from work and collapsing on the couch in exhaustion to actually wanting to get some exercise. (Believe me, it surprised me too!)

I have now been at my goal weight for the last four years and can truly say that this has been a real lifestyle change for me – I no longer even want to eat donuts and biscuits and, I am pleased to say, not a single piece of lettuce has passed through my lips in all that time.

Could this diet be the answer for you? It was for me but everyone's journey is different. Do I advise you to give it a try? Only if you want to see true results and are sick of being overweight and tired all the time.

This book will teach you how to switch your body into fat-burning mode and to get your body into optimal shape. No fuss, no fads and no more cabbage diets – ever!

Chapter 1:
What is the Ketogenic Diet?

Simply put, the ketogenic diet is a high fat and low carbohydrate diet, in which the dieter maintains adequate amounts of protein intake.

In medicine, the ketogenic diet, sometimes called the "keto" diet, is often used to treat refractory or hard to manage epilepsy in children.

Due to the low intake of carbohydrates required for the diet, the body discontinues the process of turning carbohydrates into glucose for energy, and produces ketones in the liver as an energy source instead.

In this chapter, we will take a more detailed look at what the ketogenic diet is all about, and where it all began.

What Does the Ketogenic Diet Do?

In a typical person's body, one who is ingesting balanced amounts of fats, carbohydrates and proteins, the body produces glucose and insulin when that person consumes something that is high in carbohydrates. Glucose is the body's go-to energy source, so to speak, because it is the easiest molecule for the body to convert into and use as energy.

Insulin is produced to help absorb the glucose into the bloodstream. Since in this case, the body is using glucose as a primary source of energy, it stores fat, which is not needed.

When one lowers their calorie, the body is forced to go into a state called ketosis. Ketosis begins naturally when the body senses that food intake is low, and is a survival tactic. When the body is in this state, it produces ketones, which are made by breaking down the fats in the liver.

When it comes to the ketogenic diet, the aim is to maintain levels of carbohydrates, fats and protein in a way that induces the metabolic state of ketosis. Ketosis is not only triggered by a lack of calories, rather it can also be cause by a lack of carbohydrates. The human body is built to adapt to a wide range of conditions for survival. This means that when you change what you put into your body, by eating more fats and completely eliminating carbohydrates, the body will turn to ketones a the main energy source.

The ketogenic diet copies the effects of fasting, which allows the body to produce ketones and ultimately end fat instead of carbohydrates. The diet maintains enough protein in order to promote growth and repair in the body. The ketogenic diet also allows enough calories in total so that one can maintain a healthy weight for their given age and height.

In the typical ketogenic diet, the ratio of fat to carbohydrates and proteins combined is four to one. Some examples of high fat foods are butter, cream, lard, olive oil and duck fat. Examples of foods that are extremely high in carbohydrates and should be avoided are grains, bread, pasta, sugar and starchy foods. Later in this book, we will discuss examples of ketogenic friendly meals.

A Brief History of the Ketogenic Diet

As mentioned above, the ketogenic diet first emerged as a treatment for epilepsy in the 1920s and 1930s. At the time, the only therapy for epilepsy which had shown any success at the time was fasting.

The ketogenic diet was developed as an alternative to this, but soon it was abandoned as a method of treatment because of the introduction of new therapies. Most cases of epilepsy could be controlled well using the new prescription drugs that were being developed, yet about twenty to thirty percent of epileptics were still not seeing results.

The ketogenic diet was reintroduced as an option for these patients, especially children.

For thousands of years, fasting has been known as a way to treat disease by ancient Greek and Indian doctors. In the Hippocratic Corpus, the treatise entitled "On the Sacred Disease", a descriptive account of the ways in which changing one's diet can help to manage epilepsy is offered. In addition, the same author relates an account of a man who was cured of epilepsy after choosing to abstain completely from food or drink.

In 1911 in France, the first modern scientific examination of fasting as a treatment for epilepsy was conducted. By this time, doctors turned to potassium bromide in order to curb seizures in patients, but this prescription proved to have negative effects on the cognitive function of patients.

For the purpose of the study, twenty patients suffering from epilepsy followed a low calorie, vegetarian diet in combination with fasting.

While many of the patients in the group were not able to maintain the dietary restrictions, two showed clear improvement in their conditions, and others showed an improvement in their mental abilities when compared to the effects of taking potassium bromide.

Meanwhile, the dawn of the twentieth century in America found Bernarr Macfadden making the idea of fasting for the benefit of one's health a popular one.

His student, Hugh Conklin, focused specifically on what fasting could do for epilepsy as well. Coklin though that epileptic seizures were the result of a substance produced in the intestine and that fasting for a period of 18 to 25 days would allow time for the toxin to dissipate. In order to verify his theory, Conklin prescribed a water diet for his epileptic patients.

His reports showed ninety percent of children and fifty percent of adults to be completely cured by this. Later, the study was analyzed and it was revealed that twenty percent of his patients were free of their seizures completely, while fifty percent did show some improvement. With this information, fasting as therapy for epilepsy soon became a mainstream practice.

In 1921, Rollin Woodyatt, and endocrinologist, found that as a result of starvation, the liver produced three water soluble compounds: acetone, β-hydroxybutyrate and acetoacetate. Together, these compounds make up ketone bodies and Woodyatt also found that if a person followed a diet that was rich in fat and low in carbohydrates, they would be subjected to the same effect. The same year, Russel Wilder from the Mayo Clinic coined the term "ketogenic diet" and began to effectively use it as a treatment for epilepsy.

Chapter 2:
Ketosis: Facts and Myths

In the previous chapter, we discussed the process of ketosis and what part it plays in the ketogenic diet. There are a lot of misconceptions about how ketosis works, what causes it and what risks are associated with ketosis. In this chapter, we will address some of the myths that are commonly stated about ketosis, as well as specific facts about the process.

What is Ketosis?

Ketosis is a metabolic process which is completely normal. It is something that our body does in order to continue to function properly in a variety of situations. When the body does not have enough carbohydrates from food to convert into energy for cell function, it begins to burn fat instead. The process of the body burning fat creates ketones.

For someone who is eating a healthy and well balanced diet, the body is able to easily control how much fat it burns, and thus does not produce or use ketones. However, in the absence of one of two things, either calories or carbs (or both), the body will switch to using the process of ketosis in order to gain energy.

Ketosis can also take place during pregnancy, or after an extended period of physical exertion or exercise. People who suffer from diabetes which is not controlled may also experience ketosis as a result of not using enough insulin.

Ketosis is the way that the body powers itself normally as we sleep. It was also a common process in our primitive ancestors who survived on a high protein, high fat and low carbohydrate diet. For instance, the Native American Indians of the Northern Plains and northern Eskimos rely heavily on this process because of the restricted amounts of carbohydrates occurring naturally in their diets.

The Dangers of Ketoacidosis

Ketoacidosis is a condition that can be fatal if not checked in time. It is commonly seen in persons who have Type 1 diabetes and insulin dependent Type 2 diabetes. Ketoacidosis is not the same as normal dietary ketosis, which does not pose such fatal risks.

In diabetics, the abnormally low levels of insulin that naturally occur in the body can lead to a buildup of glucose in the blood which can become toxic when insulin levels are not properly controlled. This is because the glucose cannot enter the cells to produce energy without the help of insulin. This causes excessive urination, thirst and dehydration.

Even though there may be more than enough glucose within the blood stream, the body has no way to use any of it for energy, so of course, it must turn to breaking down fat and muscle tissues for energy sources.

Ketoacidosis takes place when there is excessively high levels of glucose and ketones in the body at the same time. This combination causes the chemical makeup of the blood, specifically its pH to change, lowering to levels that are unhealthy. The body relies heavily on the maintenance of a balanced pH in order to function, so when the makeup changes as radically as it does in the event of ketoacidosis, the results can be life threatening.

Ketoacidosis will never occur in someone who is not diabetic and chooses to abide by a low carbohydrate diet.

Normal dietary ketosis will keep blood glucose levels stable and within a healthy range. It also prevents the breakdown of healthy muscle tissue which occurs excessively during ketoacidosis. In addition, because the individual's carbohydrate intake is restricted, there is no buildup of excess glucose.

In fact, the blood glucose level will remain completely stable in a non-diabetic individual practicing the ketogenic diet.

5 Common Myths About Ketosis

In spite of the scientific evidence of the benefits that a ketogenic diet can have on one's general health, there is a lot of misunderstanding about the ways in which keeping to a restricted carbohydrate diet can affect the body, either negatively or positively.

In this section, we will discuss some of the common misconceptions about ketosis and how it can affect the body and debunk them.

Myth #1: If You Do Not Eat Carbs, You Cannot Be Healthy

Many individuals believe that carbohydrates are a necessary nutrient for good health. Although it was once commonly believed that carbohydrates were necessary to provide glucose which would fuel the brain and prevent hypoglycemia, this is an old way of thinking. Essential nutrients are nutrients that the body cannot produce and thus can only get through you ingesting them on a regular basis.

While essential proteins and essential fatty acids exist, an essential carbohydrate is nonexistent. When the body is in ketosis, glucose is saved so that whatever amounts of glucose present enter the blood stream from the restricted amounts of carbohydrates ingested in a low carbohydrate diet.

Once the body fully becomes adapted to using ketosis, the brain begins to use ketones for more than half of the energy that the body and it needs, and less glucose is necessary as ketones step in as an alternative fuel method.

The liver can actually generate the small amount of glucose that is needed for brain fuel from glycogen which is stored there. If necessary, the body can also make glucose from protein which is in your food. This means that carbohydrates are not essential nutrients.

A clear representation of this fact is that, as mentioned before, the Inuit people of Alaska and others such as the Masai of Africa live without eating carbohydrates for extended periods of time without experiencing any negative effects on health and well-being.

Myth #2: too Much Protein Will Result in Kidney Damage

Another common untruth about low carbohydrate diets are that the kidneys will sustain damage from the high amounts of protein that are consumed in place of carbohydrates.

Low carb diets do not necessarily mean the same thing as high protein diets. The absent carbohydrates in a low carbohydrate diet is replaced with healthy fats. In the ketogenic diet, there is only a need for moderate consumption of protein.

There is a lot of research that shows that people who are healthy and do not have a history of kidney disease can eat a little extra protein with no harmful effects to their general health or kidney health.

One study which was published in September of 2005 conducted by William F. Martin and Nancy Rodriquez of the University of Connecticut Department of Nutritional Sciences, and Lawrence E. Armstrong of the University Of Connecticut Department Of Kinesiology examined the effects of increased protein take in the general public due to the weight loss diet trends of the time.

This study was conducted specifically to provide a response to the question of whether or not it is safe to make a habit of consuming more protein that is recommended.

The study concluded with the finding that there is no significant evidence that there are negative effects of high intakes of protein on kidney function in persons who are healthy.

Myth #3: A Low Carbohydrate Diet Will Lead to Osteoporosis

This myth is connected to the idea that the ketogenic diet is synonymous with a high protein diet, which again is not necessarily the case. The ketogenic is a high fat and moderate protein diet. With this in mind, it is essential to consume protein to maintain good bone health.

In addition to the presence of calcium and vitamin D, proteins are one of the key nutrients when it comes to preventing osteoporosis.

As a matter of fact, patients who have suffered hip fractures are often noted to have had low protein intakes. Also, a deficient amount of protein in one's diet can cause bone mass and strength to deteriorate and that there is an evident correlation between higher protein and stronger and denser bones.

Bone loss has actually been linked to a variety of things, including deficiency in magnesium, overconsumption of fructose, consuming too much grain while suffering from gluten intolerance, and consumption of vegetable oil.

Myth #4: A Ketogenic Diet Will Cause Heart Disease

The biggest myth associated with ketogenic diets are that the high amounts of fat that replace carbohydrates in this regimen can cause clogged arteries and heart disease. This misconception stems from the idea that saturated fat and cholesterol are the cause of heart disease.

On the contrary, studies have shown that a low carbohydrate diet can actually improve heart disease markers in comparison to other kinds of diets. In addition, a ketogenic diet specifically has been shown to have positive effects on blood tests that indicate heart disease.

There are several studies which confirm that a diet high in carbohydrates and high levels of blood sugar and insulin which result from this kind of diet are linked to inflammatory heart disease.

The more carbohydrates you ingest, the more cholesterol your body will produce. Cholesterol is a byproduct of glucose metabolism.

Myth #5: Low Carbohydrate Diets Result in Muscle Deterioration

The opposite of this is actually true: low carbohydrate diets allow for better preservation and even increasing of lean muscle mass.

A study published in 1984 by a team of scientists from MIT and Harvard University investigated two groups of women who were categorized as overweight. One group of women was placed on a low carbohydrate diet, while the other was put on a high carbohydrate diet.

Both diets allowed the women to consume up to 700 calories each day. Even with this severe caloric deficit, the larger amount of protein that was consumed by those women on the low carbohydrate diet in combination with the effects of ketosis showed a larger amount of retained muscle mass for those test subjects on the low carbohydrate diet.

Chapter 3:

Safety Check: Is the Ketogenic Diet Right for Me?

Now that you have a good foundation of basic knowledge about ketosis and the ketogenic diet, you may be ready to take the plunge and try it out. Based on what we have discussed so far, it is very unlikely that you have anything to lose by giving the ketogenic diet a try.

However, as with any diet there can be some risks involved depending on a variety of factors. In this chapter, we will examine how you can be sure that the ketogenic diet is a safe option for you.

Possible Risks Associated with the Ketogenic Diet

In the last chapter, we discussed in detail the risks associated with ketoacidosis. As a reminder, this condition in which the pH of the blood becomes overly acidic due to high levels of both ketones and glucose in the bloodstream can be very dangerous and cause serious illness in almost no time at all.

Nevertheless, this condition is largely only likely to be present in individuals who suffer from diabetes.

This means that **if you are diabetic**, you should check with your primary care physician in order to make sure that it is safe for you to try the ketogenic diet.

Some studies show that the ketogenic diet can actually help to minimize some negative symptoms linked to diabetes. One such symptom is diabetic neuropathy, which is nerve damage that is caused by diabetes.

Again, however, double check with your doctor before undertaking any dietary changes such as those required to stick with the ketogenic diet in order to ensure that your insulin levels are being properly controlled.

If you are interested in trying the ketogenic diet, you should also be aware of some harmful methods that are promoted by some in order to undertake this dietary lifestyle. Some dieters choose to try the feeding tube method of the ketogenic diet, which is frankly, extreme.

In this method, individuals stick to an 800 calorie per day diet that is high in protein and includes absolutely no carbohydrates. These calories are consumed through a feeding tube inserted into the esophagus through the nose. The only things that can be consumed in addition the liquid diet are black coffee, tea or water.

While this method will lead to rapid weight loss and some profess to have been able to keep the weight off for up to a year after, this is not the best approach to the ketogenic diet.

It should be used as a last resort, for instance in someone who is on a ventilator or suffering the ill effects that come from cancer or a stroke. In an individual who is healthy otherwise, this method can create dire complications, especially if the tube becomes contaminated, as this can lead to a serious infection.

Underlying kidney or liver issues can cause the ketogenic diet to be dangerous for some. While in the last chapter, we debunked the myth that ketosis would cause harm to one's kidneys, these studies were conducted on individuals who had no outstanding health problems.

If you struggle with liver or kidney ailments, it is probably best to check with your physician before choosing to undertake the ketogenic diet.

Proven Health Benefits of the Ketogenic Diet

Now that we have taken a clear look at the possible dangers (for some) when it comes to trying the ketogenic diet without the proper guidance of a health care professional, let's take a look at some of the benefits that the ketogenic diet can offer for most.

Hopefully, this will help you to make a decision about whether this is the right diet plan for you to pursue.

Curbs Your Appetite

One of the main reasons for many people being opposed to dieting and giving up shortly after beginning a new diet plan is hunger.

This is something that makes the ketogenic diet stand out above the rest.

Eating a lower amount of carbohydrates leads to an automatically reduced appetite.

Studies consistently prove that people who cut carbohydrate consumption and replace carbohydrates with more proteins and fats eat a lot less calories.

More Overall Weight Loss

Cutting down on carbohydrates is one of the most effective ways to lose weight.

People on low carbohydrate diets lose weight faster than those on low fat diets. This is because low carbohydrate diets help the body to shed weight from excess water. After insulin levels drop, the kidneys get rid of excess sodium, and this leads to fast weight loss within the first week or two of adhering to the ketogenic diet.

Some experts say that due to this, the ketogenic diet is not a sustainable weight loss method. However, this is not the case.

When people begin to regain lost weight after a few months of the ketogenic diet, it is usually because they have given up on sticking to the proper regimen and returned to eating the same way that they did previously.

This is why it is necessary to view the ketogenic diet as a lifestyle, rather than a fad diet, or a quick way to shed a few pounds. In order to make it work for you in the long term, you have to stick to it.

When following the ketogenic diet, a larger proportion of the fat lost will be shed in the abdominal area. It is no secret that the areas of the body in which fat are stored are what determines whether that fat will put us at risk of disease and the proportions of its negative impact on our health.

There is subcutaneous fat, or fat that is stored beneath the skin, and visceral fat, which is stored in the abdominal cavity. Visceral fat is dangerous as it tends to build up around the organs.

Having too much visceral fat can lead to inflammation, resistance to insulin - and it is believed that this kind of fat is mostly responsible for the metabolic issues experienced by the majority of people in Western society today.

When it comes to getting rid of harmful abdominal fat, low carbohydrate diets are great. They cause more overall fat loss than low fat diets, as mentioned, and most of the fat that is lost comes from the abdominal cavity. Over time, this will lead to a highly reduced risk of succumbing to type 2 diabetes and heart disease.

Helps to Balance Cholesterol

Most people find it hard to believe that a ketogenic diet can actually reduce cholesterol levels, especially because it contains such a high percentage of fats and saturated fats. That is because the media has previously vilified fats, particularly saturated fats.

Scientific research is, however, now pointing to the fact that it is, in fact, the low-fat diets that are more problematic in this regard, especially as our understanding of cholesterol increases.

Previously, it was thought that all cholesterol was bad and that raised cholesterol levels were a risk factor for heart disease and other lifestyle diseases. Then science discovered that there were actually two types of lipoproteins that transported cholesterol around the body – Low Density Lipoprotein and High Density Lipoprotein.

Now, and this is important, LDL is what is responsible for plaque building up in your arteries. The particle size is smaller and more easily able to pass through the blood barrier and so an excess of LDL stored in the body's tissues can be dangerous to your health.

HDL, on the other hand, has a very big particle size and is less likely to be able to cross over into the blood stream when stored in the body's fatty tissues. In addition, these molecules act like a magnet to roving LDL particles and mop them up.

What this means, in essence, is that the traditional cholesterol count is simply not an accurate measure of how healthy you are – you can have low or normal cholesterol levels and, if it is primarily LDL, you could still have a problem. You need to check your levels of HDL and LDL cholesterol.

Initially, your overall cholesterol levels will increase on a ketogenic diet but this will level off in time as the HDL starts to replace the LDL cholesterol.

Chapter 4:

The 3 Basic Principles of a Ketogenic Diet Plan

With all of the complex information that you have learned about the ketogenic diet so far, it may seem that following the diet itself is even more complicated. However, this is far from the case. In order to successfully incorporate the ketogenic diet into your lifestyle, there are only a few basic guidelines that you have to follow. Once you stick to the three basic principles of a ketogenic diet plan, which we will discuss in this chapter, you will be able to easily make the ketogenic diet a part of your life.

The following guidelines are where to start when planning your ketogenic diet plan. You will need to monitor your progress and may need to adjust your food intake in order to achieve full ketosis. As you lose weight, you will also need to rethink what you are eating.

Fat: 60 to 75 percent of calories

Protein: 15 to 30 percent of calories

Carbohydrates: 5 to 10 percent of calories

We will go over how to work out the overall allowed calorie count per day in a later chapter.

Low Carb

Unlike the conception that most people have of the ketogenic diet, the diet does involve some carbohydrate consumption.

The key is that the amount of carbohydrates that you are eating must be limited in order for ketosis to begin so that you can experience the benefits of the diet, which begin with that metabolic process.

Moderate Protein

Low carb diets like the Atkins Diet allow you to eat as much fat and protein as you want.

The theory is that because fat and protein are so filling, you will automatically eat less.

This is not in accordance with true ketogenic principles because eating too much protein can interfere with achieving ketogenesis.

Higher Fat

You will be eating a lot more fat on this diet and this may scare some people initially. I have gallstones and I was certain that the increased fat intake would play merry havoc with me - normally when you eat foods too high in fat when you have gallstones, you end up having a very painful episode.

What surprised me is that I did not battle with this at all so I did a little more research.

It turns out that it is not so much about the quantity as the quality of the fat that you consume.

Trans-fatty acids are one of the unhealthiest substances in our food today and are present in many processed foods. These fats are nothing short of toxic and provide little of the nourishment that the body needs.

I can still hear some people thinking about the high fat content of this diet and that is understandable - after all, it is about double what the recommended daily allowance for fat is.

What we need to keep in mind is that fat is now being used as fuel for our bodies instead of as a backup in case the glucose runs out - you will need more fat to replace the carbs that you have cut out.

What to Eat While on the Ketogenic Diet

While you have many options in terms of what to eat when you are adhering to the guidelines of the ketogenic diet, there are a few foods that you will do well to avoid all together.

These foods offer no nutritional value, and directly oppose the aims of the ketogenic diet.

In this section, we will discuss a few foods that you should try your best to stay away from in order to reap the most reward from following the ketogenic diet.

We will also look at the kinds of foods that it is okay for you to eat from time to time, and those which you can eat as much as you want.

Foods to Avoid

Some foods that you should avoid completely include those that are rich in carbohydrates. Remember, one of the main principles of the ketogenic diet are consuming a low amount of carbs in order to push the body into a state of ketosis.

Consuming foods that are high in carbohydrates will defeat this purpose entirely, and will certainly be the cause of a lack of progress down the line.

One should also stay away from meat that is not organic, also known as factory-farmed meat, and processed foods.

Factory farmed meat is often associated with harmful hormones and steroids that are fed to the animals as a part of their regular diet in order to promote faster development, and thus larger profits for the establishment farming them.

These can be harmful when ingested by humans, causing subtle changes in the body that compile over time.

That said, if buying organic produce is not within your budget, you can still benefit from following a ketogenic diet.

Processed foods have often been stripped completely of their nutritional value, and offer nothing but empty calories, which is why these should be avoided at all costs as well.

Here is a short list of foods that may fall into these categories. Of course, not every food that you may encounter is on this list, but based on this information and the principles discussed earlier in this chapter, you should be able to deduce whether or not a type of food falls into the category of foods to avoid.

1) All grains.

   This includes whole grains, such as wheat, rye, corn, barley, bulgur, oats, rice, buckwheat, sprouted grains, sorghum and amaranth.

   You should also stay away from quinoa and even white potatoes. Products that include grains in anyway should also be avoided. Some of these are pasta, bread, pizza, cookies and crackers.

2) Sugar and Sweets.

   Consuming too much sugar and sweets will be counteractive to the process of ketosis by necessitating a large amount of glucose in order to metabolize the sugar added to the blood stream.

   This means that one should avoid things such as high fructose corn syrup, table sugar, agave syrup and things that have a high sugar content such as ice cream, cake, sweet pudding, and sugary soft drinks or sodas.

3) Factory farmed meats, such as pork and fish.

Factory farmed meats have high levels of omega 6 fatty acids. Farmed fish specifically can contain PCBs or polychlorinated biphenyls, which have been found to cause several harmful effects to human health. High levels of PCBs can cause problems in the immune system and in liver function. PCBs can also cause cancer, specifically of the liver. Fish that are high in mercury should be avoided as well.

4) Processed foods.

These include foods that feature additives and preservatives such as carrageenan, monosodium glutamate (MSG), sulphites, Bisphenol A (BPA) and wheat gluten.

5) Refined fats and oils such as sunflower oil, safflower oil, cottonseed oil, canola oil, soybean oil, grapeseed oil and corn oil. One should also avoid artificial fats such as margarine.

6) Products that are advertised as "low-fat", "low-carb" and "zero-carb". These products may feature high carbohydrate contents or artificial additives. These include diet sodas and drinks and sugar free chewing gum.

7) Artificial sweeteners such as Splenda and Equal, or any other sweetener that contains aspartame, acesulfame, sucralose or saccharin.

These products can lead to uncontrollable cravings among other problems, in the long term.

8) Milk.

If necessary, small amounts of raw, full fat milk is allowed. However, milk is not recommended for many reasons. One of these is that milk is not easy to digest, due to the fact that through the process of pasteurization the "good bacteria" that would aid in digestion is absent. Milk may also contain hormones. In addition, milk has a fairly high carbohydrate content. It has about four or five grams of carbohydrate for every 100 milliliters.

9) Tropical Fruit, High Carb Fruit, Fruit Juices and Dried Fruits.

These include but are not limited to fruits such as pineapples, mangoes, bananas, papayas, tangerines, grapes, dates and raisins. Fruit juices have a very high sugar content, and are missing many of the nutrients that can be reaped from consuming whole fruits.

Foods to Eat Occasionally

There are many foods that you can consume while on the ketogenic diet, but that should be consumed in limited quantities for one reason or another.

The exact limits that you will have to adhere to when it comes to these foods is based entirely on your individual carb limit, which of course will be based on your body, its needs and your overall goals. Here is a brief list of some of these foods in each of the basic food groups.

1) Vegetables, Mushrooms and Fruits.

   Some vegetables and fruits that you should try to limit your consumption of are cruciferous vegetables, such as white and green cabbage, cauliflower, broccoli, red cabbage, Brussel sprouts, fennel, turnips and rutabaga. You should also limit the amount of nightshades you eat. Nightshades are vegetables like eggplant, tomato and pepper. Certain root vegetables can be very starchy and should be kept to a minimum as well. These include but are not limited to spring onions, leeks, garlic, onions, mushrooms, and squash.

   Sea vegetables such as nori and Kombu, as well as okra, bean sprouts, sugar snap peas, wax beans, artichokes and water chestnuts should be consumed in limited amounts.

Some fruits that you should keep an eye on while eating include berries, like blackberries, strawberries, raspberries, cranberries, mulberries, rhubarb and olives.

2) Grain-fed animal sources and full- fat Dairy.

Earlier in this chapter, we noted that factory farmed meat and milk should be avoided as much as possible. However, one is not banned from animal sources altogether on the ketogenic diet.

Things like beef, poultry, eggs and ghee can be eaten from time to time.

Dairy products such as plain full fat yogurt, cream, sour cream, cheese and cottage cheese can also be eaten.

Nevertheless, you should take care to avoid dairy products which are labeled low fat, as many of these have high amounts of starch and sugar.

Bacon can also be consumed in small amounts, however make sure that you are aware of any existence of preservatives and added starch in the bacon that you choose to consume, as both of these are things that you should avoid at all costs.

3) Nuts and Seeds.

Nuts and seeds are good for you and especially offer a lot of heart benefits. You can eat macadamia nuts, which are very low in carbs and high in omega 3s, occasionally. Other nuts that you can consume in limited amounts are pecans, almonds, walnuts, hazelnuts, pine nuts, pumpkin seeds, sunflower seeds, flaxseed, sesame seeds, hemp seeds and Brazil nuts.

4) Fermented Soy Products and Condiments.

If you should choose to indulge in soy products, which is not recommended due to the many negative health effects associated with soy, you should only consume non-genetically modified soy products which have been fermented. Some examples of these are Natto, Tempeh, soy sauce and paleo friendly coconut aminos. You can also eat limited amounts of edamame and unprocessed black soybeans.

When it comes to condiments, you should try to avoid any sweeteners that are labeled as "zero-carb", but should you need a sweetener, consume these only in small amounts. You should also eat limited amounts of thickeners such as arrowroot powder and xanthan gum.

Sugar free tomato products like sugar free tomato puree, passata and ketchup should be avoided as well, as cocoa, carob powder and extra dark chocolate due to the high content of soy lecithin. Sugar free chewing gums and mints should be eaten with care, as some of them may contain carbs.

5) Vegetables, Fruits, Nuts and Seeds with Average Levels of Carbohydrates and Alcohol.

Some foods that do not have low carbohydrate levels can be okay to eat from time to time, based on your individual daily carb limit. Some of these are celery, carrots, beets, parsnips and sweet potato. Some may also be able to enjoy small amounts of watermelon, cantaloupe, honeydew melons, pistachios, cashews and chestnuts. While you can eat small amounts of apricots, dragon fruit, peaches, nectarines, apples, grapefruits, kiwis, oranges, plums, cherries, figs and pears, should be avoided completely if at all possible. When it comes to alcohol, during the stage of the diet during which you are trying to lose weight, you should avoid all alcohol. However, once you have reached weight maintenance, you can enjoy small amounts of dry red and white wine and unsweetened spirits.

Foods to Eat to Your Heart's (and Stomach's) Content

This list of foods that you cannot enjoy while on the ketogenic diet probably seems endless. However, there are several delicious foods that you can enjoy and in this section we will discuss them in each of their food groups.

1) Grass-fed and wild animal sources.

   In the context of animal products, you can enjoy grass-fed meat such as beef, lamb, goat and venison, as well as wild caught fish and seafood. Pastured pork and poultry is also okay to eat, as well as pastured eggs, gelatin, ghee and butter. Be mindful of sausages and meat with breadcrumb coating, as well as hot dogs and meat that comes doused in sugary or starchy sauce, as these should be avoided at all costs. Grass fed organ meats are also okay, and offer lots of nutritional value.

2) Healthy Fats.

   These include saturated fat, such as that which makes up lard, tallow, duck fat, goose fat, chicken fat, butter, clarified butter or ghee and coconut oil. Mono-unsaturated fats are also allowed without limit, and these can be found in foods such as avocado, macadamia nuts and olive oil. You can also enjoy polyunsaturated omega 3s, especially those from animal sources such as fish and seafood.

3) Non Starchy Vegetables.

Leafy greens such as Swiss chard, bok choy, lettuce, chard, spinach, chives, endive and radicchio have many health benefits and can be eaten as much as you please. Some cruciferous vegetables such as kale, kohlrabi and radishes are allowed, in addition to celery stalks, asparagus, cucumber, summer squash (such as zucchini and spaghetti squash) and bamboo shoots.

4) Beverages and Condiments.

In terms of beverages and condiments, there are a few that you can enjoy with abandon. Some beverages that you can feel free to indulge in whenever you please are water, black coffee or coffee with cream or coconut milk, and black or herbal tea. In order to add dimension to your meals, you are allowed to eat unlimited amounts of several types of condiments. These include pork rinds, which can be used for breading in place of panko or bread crumbs, mayonnaise, mustard, pesto, pickles, fermented foods like kimchi and sauerkraut and homemade bone broth. All spices and herbs are also allowed as well as lemon juice, lime juice and zest from both of these fruits.

Whey protein without additives, artificial sweeteners, hormones and soy lecithin, egg whites and gelatin from grass fed and hormone free animals can also be eaten.

The Matter of Substitutes

Many of the foods that you are likely accustomed to eating on a daily basis currently are not allowed as part of a strict ketogenic diet. Does this mean that you will no longer be able to enjoy the taste of your favorite foods? This is not necessarily the case. There are many options when it comes to substituting your favorite foods and ingredients with ketogenic diet friendly foods. In this section, we will take a look at what foods or meals you can use to replace for those high carbohydrate favorites.

Breakfast

For your favorite breakfast foods, there are lots of low carb options that are just as delicious, if not more so. For example, try switching out flavored yogurt with full fat Greek yogurt or coconut milk yogurt. You can also try having full fat cottage cheese or sour cream instead. For added flavor, mix in a few toasted nuts, berries or your favorite spices.

For your favorite breakfast cereal, substitute chia pudding, flax granola or toasted nuts.

You can also try eating salted caramel pork rind cereal, or mixed nuts that have been toasted so that they are crushed and crispy.

When it comes to oatmeal, a great replacement can be chia seed oatmeal or flaxseed oatmeal. You can even use cauliflower to get a delicious "oatmeal". Pancakes and waffles can be made with different ingredients for a lower carbohydrate version. For example, try cream cheese pancakes or almond flour waffles instead!

Dinner

What about those iconic dinner meals that have become time tested favorites, but are loaded with carbohydrates? For those, we have low carbohydrate alternatives as well. For example, instead of having a burger and French fries, have a medium sized steak with butter on it and broccoli (or cheesy broccoli) on the side. If steak is not your thing, or a little bit ambitious for your budget, try a burger without a bun or use vegetables for buns.

For pizza, have a pizza with an alternative crust. One great example of this is a crust made with almond flour. You can add cheese to the crust for a little bit of extra indulgence, and you will not even know the difference when compared to a traditional pizza crust.

Fried Chicken is another comfort food that can be made just as good, if not better, with low carbohydrate options. Try using pork rinds that have been ground up in a food processor and adding parmesan cheese to it. This will give you the fried chicken you love, with a crispy crust and a moist and juicy inside.

For your favorite canned soup, make soups yourself using fresh ingredients, including fresh cream as a base. Try making your favorite soup in bulk and freezing it for quick and easy meals when you need them. In order to replace your favorite pasta, which is a deadly food in terms of the ketogenic diet, meaning it is absolutely jam packed with carbohydrates, why not try Zoodles? These are noodles made of zucchini which you can cover with your favorite cream sauce.

Chapter 5:

The Most Famous Ketogenic Diet in History

Now that we have covered the basics concerning the ketogenic diet, let us also go over what some people consider the most famous ketogenic diet in history – the Atkins Diet. Originally developed in the 1970's, this diet has become very popular. Whilst not the first diet based on ketogenic principles, it was the first such diet specifically targeted at weight loss.

Prior to this, strict ketogenic diets had been employed but generally only as a therapeutic treatment for epilepsy. In fact, until the "Atkins Revolution" started, these diets had fallen by the wayside as it was felt that pharmaceuticals could better address the issue.

Now, please note that I say ketogenic-based diet when referring to the Atkin's Diet. Whilst they are very similar, they are not exactly the same at all. Whilst the aim of both is that you achieve a ketogenic state, they go about this quite differently.

With a true ketogenic diet, you have a lot more freedom in terms of what you are able to incorporate into your diet but you have to be a lot stricter when it comes to protein intake.

The Atkin's Diet is a lot stricter when it comes to what you may and may not eat but does not place nearly as much emphasis on limiting your protein intake. Essentially, a strict ketogenic diet can be compared to the induction phase of the Atkin's diet.

So, which one is better overall? The simple truth is that both diets will work to some degree but if you want to fast-track your success, you will need to keep tabs on what you eat.

None of us like calorie counting – it is a pain in the butt – but you also cannot expect to lose weight as efficiently as possible if you are not willing to adhere to the basic ratio of macro-nutrients as laid out in the previous chapter. The good news is that it does become a lot easier over time.

Chapter 6:
Do I Need to Calorie Count?

Now this is probably not what you want to hear but yes, you will need to do some calorie counting. It is basic science – if you want to lose weight, you need to make sure that you use more energy than you take in every day.

The good news is that this calorie counting will not feel as restrictive as it would in normal diets and that there is some scope for playing with the figures.

The following formula can give you a starting point:

Men: 10 × weight (kg) + 6.25 × height (cm) – 5 × age (y) + 5

Women: 10 × weight (kg) + 6.25 × height (cm) – 5 × age (y) – 161

You need to aim for a daily calorie deficit of 500 calories in order to lose about a pound a week. Do not go and cut the calories too drastically in the hope of losing more – cutting 500 is plenty when you combine it with the improved fat-burning ability of your body on this new plan.

With a ketogenic diet, it is important to keep the ratio of macronutrients right, in addition to monitoring your overall calorie count so it does pay to either look for an app that enables you to check what the calorie content of the food that you want to eat is.

In general though, this diet is a bit more forgiving than most if you do exceed your calorie count once in a while, as long as the food is low in carbs.

Calorie counting here is a bit annoying at first but will pay great dividends in the end. Eventually, once you get used to eating this way and what the portion sizes are, you will be able to eyeball portions and will be able to dispense with calorie counting.

If, however, your weight loss starts to slow down, you may need to implement it again just in case you are inadvertently eating more than you should.

Chapter 7:

Converting - The Secret to a Clean Break

(and Mistakes to Avoid!)

Okay, so it's time for the hard truth – for those of you waiting for the catch, here it is – switching over to a very low-carb diet may be difficult, at least at first. Basically, you are changing up the way that your body wants to do things and making it work harder in the process. This will not go over so well initially and you can expect to feel as though you have the flu while the body is making this adjustment.

The severity of the "withdrawal" symptoms and duration of this period of adjustment will differ from person to person and so it is hard to say what you will experience. The symptoms are bound to be worse for you if you went from eating a diet high in refined carbs.

My diet before consisted mainly of junk food – I used to have donuts for breakfast and wash them down with soda (Low-calorie soda, of course!) so I did have a hard time when I switched over.

Fortunately, you will likely only need to endure the symptoms for around about three to seven days or so and there is a lot that you can do to help you feel better.

I do have one word of caution here – this changeover process can take a few weeks in some cases but if you employ the methods listed below and you still feel really bad after two weeks, you may need to reconsider the diet.

For 90% of people, this diet is more in line with the way that they should be eating on a daily basis. For the remaining 10%, this diet is not going to work and can be harmful to health if followed for a protracted period.

Obviously you need to be guided by your body and you need to employ a little common sense as well. Do not schedule the first week of this diet for a particularly busy or stressful period for you. Here are ways to ensure that the transition is as easy as possible and what to try if the diet does not seem to be working for you.

Rule Number 1: Adhere To The Guidelines Strictly and Adjust When And If Necessary

Look out for the signs that your body has gone into ketosis and adjust the quantities of macronutrients as and where necessary if it is not. Sometimes even just tweaking the ratios a couple of percentage points in either direction can be the difference between failure and success.

Rule Number 2: Work Out The Ratios And Reassess As You Lose Weight

You will lose weight if you wing it but it is a lot better to take the time to actually calculate the optimal ratios. It is really that important if you are serious about making a lasting change in your life.

It does not take that long at all:

Work out the number of total calories necessary for the day and then work out the total number of carbs, proteins and fats that you can eat in terms of optimal ratios.

Carbs: You may need to do a little fine-tuning here because everyone is different. For many people, going into ketosis means staying at 5% total intake of carbs. For others, this may simply be too low. Monitor your results and see what works for you.

To work out how many carbs you are allowed, take the figure worked out above and multiply it by 5% - 10%. Take the resulting figure and divide by 4 in order to work out how many grams of carbs you should be eating on a day to day basis. (1 gram of carbs contains about 4 calories and that is why you are dividing by 4.)

You do need to be aware of the difference between total and net carbs here. You will need to work with the net carbs here. To find out what the net carbs in a particular food are, take the total carb count and subtract the total grams of fiber.

Fat: Fat is the next one to work out. Take your total calorie count and multiply it by 60% - 75%. Divide the resultant figure by 9 to get the number of grams of fat that you can eat on a daily basis. (1 gram of fat contains 9 calories.)

Protein: Whatever calorie count is left over, will need to come from protein. Multiply the overall calorie count by 15% - 20% and divide this total by 4. (1 gram of protein contains 4 calories).

Get Thee Behind Me, Banned Foods

Before you get started, go through your grocery cupboards and drawers and remove any banned foods. It is better to get temptation right out of the way, especially when you start this plan.

Avoid those aisles in the store – you know the aisles I am talking about!

What I did was to order my meat online – it got delivered to my door and to buy the rest of the produce I needed at the local, weekly farmer's market. Not only did I not have to go down Temptation Alley while queuing for my groceries, I also got much nicer produce.

If that is not an option for you, give yourself the best possible chance by planning your shopping trips carefully. Make sure that you have had a snack before going shopping – nothing blunts your common sense like feeling slightly hungry – and ensure that you make a list and only buy what is on the list. Shop when you are not under pressure and, preferably, on the quieter days of the week, like Wednesday instead of Saturday – the grocery store is bound to have more tempting freshly baked goods over the weekend than during the week.

If you are still not losing weight, or if you are not feeling great on the plan after the initial adjustment phase, one of the following may be an issue.

Mistake Number 1 – Too Many Carbs

What exactly is a low-carb diet? Look it up online and you will see that there are a whole lot of different answers but, generally speaking, carb intake of between 100 grams and 150 grams daily is considered low and it is a lot lower than what most people following a normal Western diet take in.

If you cut back to this level, you are bound to lose some weight.

But even this level is too high for attaining ketosis. In most cases you need to restrict your carb intake to less than 50 grams a day in order to kick-start ketosis.

And that means that your carb choices are very restricted – you will basically be relying on vegetable mostly and can maybe incorporate a small amount of berries. That basically translates into hardly any fruit at all.

If you are not getting the weight loss results that you require, try checking the carb content in your diet and cutting it back if necessary. In a later chapter, we will go through how you can tell if your body has gone into ketosis.

Mistake Number 2 – Too Much Protein

Protein is extremely important in our diets – we need it to help boost feelings of satiety and to rev up fat burning. In general terms, the more protein you eat, the more fat you will lose.

It would seem that there is no such thing as too much protein.

Again, it is not quite that simple – it is possible that you are hampering your efforts to get your body into ketosis by eating too much protein.

If you are eating more protein than your body can use, the amino acids in the excess will be converted to glucose. This, in turn, will prevent you from reaching full ketosis.

However, low-carb dieters who eat a lot of lean animal foods can end up eating too much of it.

No more than 20% of your total calorie intake should consist of protein.

You also need to adjust this as you lose weight. Aim for around 0.8 grams of protein for every pound of bodyweight.

Mistake Number 3 – Not Eating Enough Fat

For most people, the idea that 75% of our calorie intake from fat flies in the face of what we have been conditioned to believe in the last forty years or so.

This high level of fat is essential to the sustainability of the diet overall. Because you are removing what was probably your main source of energy – carbs – you need to replace it with something so that you do not starve.

Where a lot of people go wrong is that they think that they can combine a low-fat and low-carb diet for optimal results – as a result, they literally starve their bodies of energy and are not able to maintain the results that they would like to.

Do not underestimate your body's instinctive drive to survive. Whilst initially you might have the willpower to stick to a low-carb and low-fat diet, you will not be able to maintain it for long.

If you are on a ketogenic diet, you should never feel hungry. If you are feeling hungry there is a better than average chance that you are eating too little fat.

The key here is to eat healthy, natural fats such as saturated fats, Omega-3 fatty acids and monounsaturated fats and to avoid any trans-fats or processed fats.

What this means is that you can indulge your love of great tasting food and start cooking with butter, coconut oil and olive oils, etc.

Mistake Number 4 – Not Getting Enough Sodium

One of the reasons that a ketogenic plan works so well is that there is a big reduction when it comes to insulin in the blood stream. This is a good thing – with too much insulin in the blood stream, your body holds onto its fat stores.

The downside is that insulin also regulates the amount of sodium retained in the kidneys.

Reduce insulin levels and you will also get rid of excess water and sodium in the body.

The problem is that sodium is essential for health – whilst most of us eat too much anyway, the body does need some to survive.

It is actually this lack of sodium that results in people suffering from side effects like fatigue, constipation, headaches and dizziness.

If you find that you are suffering with these side effects, add more sodium into your diet or start drinking a daily cup of broth.

This is one of the main reasons people get side effects on low-carb diets… such as lightheadedness, fatigue, headaches and even constipation.

Chapter 8:
Breakfast Recipes

Cheesy Pancakes

Ingredients:

2 oz. full fat cream cheese

2 large eggs

1 tablespoon coconut flour

½ teaspoon powdered cinnamon

½ sachet Stevia powder

Instructions:

Beat together everything well and fry in coconut oil or ghee over a medium heat until done, in the same way as you would any other pancakes, flipping once.

Serve piping hot!

Granola Keto Style

Ingredients:

5 tablespoons flaked coconut

7 tablespoons ground Hemp seeds

5 tablespoons ground Flaxseed

2 tablespoons Psyllium husk

2 tablespoons ground Sesame seeds

2 tablespoons dark cocoa powder (no added sugar)

Instructions:

Mix together everything and refrigerate until ready to eat.

Serve with full fat cream or with a little water.

Breakfast Latte With a Difference

Ingredients:

2 cups strong, fresh, filter coffee

1 cup full fat Coconut Milk

1/4 cup Pureed Pumpkin

2 teaspoons Spice Blend for Pumpkin Pie

1/2 teaspoon powdered Cinnamon

1 teaspoon good quality Vanilla Extract

2 tablespoons double Cream

2 tablespoons farm butter

15 drops Glycerite

Instructions:

Put the milk, pumpkin, spice and butter in a pot and cook slowly until it comes to a boil.

Add the coffee and stir well.

Take off the heat and mix in the rest of the ingredients.

Blend until smooth.

French Toast to Die for

Ingredients:

4 slices low-carb bread, day old

1 egg

2 tablespoons double Cream

2 tablespoons Butter

1/8 teaspoon good quality Orange Extract

1/2 teaspoon good quality Vanilla Extract

1/4 teaspoon Pumpkin Pie Spice

Instructions:

Mix the egg, the extracts and the spice together until well-combined.

Soak each slice of bread in mixture, flip and then fry in butter as you would normal French toast.

Low-Carb Bread

Ingredients:

1 1/2 cup finely ground Almond Flour

3 large Eggs, Whites only – reserve yolks for another dish

1/2 cup full fat Coconut Milk

1/2 cup Pureed Pumpkin

1/4 cup Psyllium Powder

1/4 cup powdered Swerve

1 1/2 teaspoon Pumpkin Pie Spice

2 teaspoons Baking Powder

1/2 teaspoon Salt

Instructions:

Warm up your oven to a temperature of 350F.

Separate the dry and wet ingredients, sift all the dry ingredients and combine.

Set a ramekin filled with water on the lowest oven rack.

Mix the milk and puree together and fold into the dry ingredients.

Whisk the egg whites till soft peak stage has been reached and then fold them in as well. Mix till dough is smooth.

Spray a loaf tin with baking spray and put the dough in it. Bake for about an hour and a quarter.

Keto Waffles

Ingredients:

1 - 1 1/2 cup freshly shredded Cauliflower

1/2 cup good quality Mozzarella

1/4 cup good quality shredded Parmesan

1/2 cup good quality shredded Cheddar Cheese

3 free range Eggs

3 tablespoons snipped Chives

1/2 teaspoon Powdered Onion

1/2 teaspoon Powdered Garlic

1/4 teaspoon Flaked Chili Pepper

Seasoning as required

Instructions:

Process the cauliflower until small and crumbly.

Add in the cheeses and process until mixed.

Follow with the rest of the ingredients and process until the batter is well-combined.

Half of this mix will make one waffle – cook as you would a normal waffle.

Serve warm.

Scrumptious Keto Breakfast Muffins

Ingredients:

1 medium Egg

1/4 cup Heavy Cream

1 slice cooked Bacon (Cured, Pan-Fried, Cooked)

1 oz. Cheddar Cheese

Salt & Black Pepper (to taste)

Instructions:

Preheat oven to 350 F

In a bowl, whisk the eggs with the cream and salt and pepper.

Spread into pam sprayed muffin tins, and fill the cups 1/2 full.

Place 1 slice crumbled bacon to each muffin and then 1/2 oz. cheese on top of each muffin.

Bake for about 15-20 minutes or until slightly browned.

Add another 1/2 oz. of cheese onto each muffin and broil until cheese is slightly browned. Enjoy!

Keto Egg Porridge

Ingredients:

2 organic free-range eggs

1/3 cup organic heavy cream without food additives

2 packages NuStevia OR your preferred sweetener to taste

2 tablespoons grass-fed butter

Ground organic cinnamon to taste

Instructions:

In a small bowl add together eggs, cream and the sweetener and whisk together.

Melt the butter in a medium saucepan over medium-high heat. Lower the heat to the minimum once the butter is melted.

Combine together the egg and cream mixture.

Cook, all the time mixing along the bottom until the mixture thickens and starts curdling.

When you see the first signs of curdling, remove the saucepan immediately from the heat.

Pour the porridge in a serving bowl. Sprinkle plenty of cinnamon on top and serve immediately.

Keto Eggs Florentine

Ingredients:

1 cup washed, fresh spinach leaves

2 tablespoons freshly grated parmesan cheese

Sea salt and pepper to taste

1 tablespoon white vinegar

2 eggs

Instructions:

Cook spinach in a microwave safe bowl in microwave or steam until wilted.

Sprinkle with parmesan cheese and season to taste.

Slice into bite size pieces and place on a plate.

Heat a pan of simmering water, adding the vinegar and stir with wooden spoon to create a whirl pool.

Break an egg into the center, turn of the heat and leave covered until set (3-4 minutes).

Repeat with second egg.

Place eggs on spinach and serve.

Quick & Easy Keto Spanish Omelet

Ingredients:

3 eggs

Cayenne or black pepper

½ cup finely chopped vegetables e.g. olives, onions, chives, capsicum, parsley, spinach, zucchini.

Instructions:

In a medium pan lightly stir-fry vegetables in extra virgin olive oil and remove.

Cook eggs with one tablespoon of water and pinch of pepper.

When almost cooked top with vegetables and flip to heat through.

Keto Fetta, Zucchini and Red Capsicum Frittata

Ingredients:

2 cups coarsely chopped vegetables (Pumpkin, Zucchini, Red capsicum)

120 g fetta crumbled

3 eggs

¼ cup cream

2 tablespoons of olive oil

Instructions:

Cut and steam vegetables until tender, set aside.

Beat eggs with cream, set aside.

Add oil to a thick base fry pan and place on a very low heat.

Mix in half of egg mixture to pan, put vegetables and crumbled feta in pan and cover with remaining egg mixture.

Cover with lid and cook on very low heat until cooked through.

Place uncovered fry pan under grill until top of frittata turns golden brown.

Kristy's Ketogenic Pancakes

Ingredients:

1 scoop of KetogenX Vanilla

1 tablespoon of almond or hazelnut meal

2 tablespoons water

1 egg

Instructions:

Add together ingredients in a bowl.

In a non-stick pan, cook on moderate heat for approximately 2 to 3 minutes on each side.

(Watch carefully as it may burn quickly!)

Serve buttered with a handful of mixed berries.

Keto Morning Breakfast Tea

Ingredients:

16 ounces water

2 tea bags

1 tablespoon ghee

1 tablespoon coconut oil

1/2 teaspoon vanilla extract

No carb artificial sweetener

Instructions:

Make the tea, set aside.

In a different container melt the ghee.

Add coconut oil and vanilla to the melted ghee.

Pour tea from mug into the magic bullet cup.

Screw bottom on and blend until mixed thoroughly.

Spinach Feta Keto Muffins

Ingredients:

6 eggs

3 slices bacon, cooked

2 cups raw spinach

1 cup crumbled feta cheese

1/2 cup cheddar cheese

Salt and pepper to taste

Instructions:

Preheat oven to 350.

Wash the spinach, drain and place in a microwave safe bowl. Microwave the spinach on high for 1 minute. Set aside to cool.

Cook bacon until it is how you like it, then set aside to cool.

In a medium mixing bowl, beat the eggs together until frothy. Mix in the crumbled feta cheese and the grated cheddar cheese.

Once the spinach and bacon are cooled enough, add them to the bowl and mix until combined.

Divide the mixture evenly among the 6 muffin cups. Bake for 30-35 minutes until muffins are firm.

Keto Coconut Waffles/Pancakes

Ingredients:

Batter

1 cup Raisins

1 Tbsp ground Cinnamon

1 Tbsp Coconut Milk

1/4 cup Coconut Flour

1/4 tsp Baking Soda

1/4 tsp ground Nutmeg

4 Pastured Eggs

Topping

Coconut Oil (for cooking)

1 Banana

1 Handful of pecans

Instructions:

For the Waffles

Blend all ingredients with a hand mixer in a medium-sized mixing bowl. Preheat waffle iron to medium-high heat. Place batter into center of waffle iron to cover about 3/4 of area for about 3–5 minutes.

For the topping

Heat coconut oil in a nonstick frying pan on medium heat. Slice banana and add to frying pan. Cook banana slices until brown and crispy on the bottom side, then flip. Add pecans to frying pan and lightly toast with the seared banana slices. Top over waffles or pancakes and serve.

Keto Breakfast Quiche Lorraine

Ingredients:

Crust

1 1/2 cups blanched almond flour

1 1/2 cups freshly grated Parmesan cheese

1/4 teaspoon Celtic sea salt

1 egg

Swiss Sauce

1 Tablespoon butter

1/2 cup chicken/beef broth

1 cup grated Swiss cheese

4 ounce cream cheese

1 teaspoon Celtic sea salt

Filling

12 slices bacon

Cheese Sauce (from above)

1/3 cup minced leeks

4 eggs, beaten

3/4 teaspoon sea salt

1/8 teaspoon cayenne pepper

Instructions:

Preheat the oven to 325 degrees F.

For the tart shell

Add together the flour, cheese and salt and mix well. Combine the egg and mix until the dough is well combined and stiff. Press pie crust into pie dish or tart pan.

Bake the crust for 12-15 minutes, or until it starts to lightly brown.

To make the Cheese Sauce

Melt butter in a medium saucepan over medium heat. Add in the rest of the ingredients and mix; season with the salt and pepper.

Meanwhile, place bacon in a large skillet, and fry over medium-high heat until crisp. Drain on paper towels, then slice coarsely. Spread bacon, into pastry shell.

In a medium bowl, whisk together cheese sauce, leeks, eggs, salt and cayenne pepper. Pour mixture into pastry shell.

Bake 15 minutes in the preheated oven.

Reduce heat to 300 degrees F and bake an additional 30 minutes, or until a knife inserted 1 inch from edge comes out clean.

Let cool and enjoy!

Keto Fluffy Coconut Flour Pancakes

Ingredients:

1/2 cup coconut flour

3 tablespoon granulated erythritol

1/2 teaspoon baking powder

1/2 teaspoon salt

6 large eggs, lightly beaten

1/4 cup butter, melted

1 cup almond milk

1/2 teaspoon vanilla extract

Additional butter or oil for the pan

Instructions:

Preheat oven to 200F.

In a large bowl, beat together coconut flour, erythritol, baking powder, and salt.

In a medium bowl, beat together eggs, melted butter, almond milk and vanilla extract.

Combine the egg mixture to the coconut flour mixture and mix well.

Heat a large skillet over medium high heat and brush with vegetable oil or melted butter.

Pour two heaping tablespoons of batter onto skillet and spread into a 3 to 4 inch circle.

Repeat until you can't fit any more pancakes into the skillet.

Cook until bottom is golden brown and top is set around the edges.

Flip carefully and continue to cook until second side is golden brown.

Remove from pan and serve warm.

Keto Ham and Swiss Frittatas

Ingredients:

1/2 lb. ham, cubed

1/2 lb. swiss cheese, cubed

1 Tablespoon Fresh rosemary, chopped

4 large whole eggs

1 1/4 cups cream, heavy whipping

2 Tablespoon dijon mustard, whole grain

Salt and fresh cracked pepper, to taste

Instructions:

Pre-heat oven to 400 F.

In a mixing bowl, stir together your bacon, ham, Swiss cheese and chopped rosemary.

Spray non-stick spray on muffin pan and then divide the mixture evenly among the muffin cups.

In the same mixing bowl, beat together your eggs, cream, mustard and a small amount of salt and pepper.

Evenly pour the egg mixture into each cup.

Bake for about 20 minutes, or until puffy and golden brown.

]Remove from oven and let rest for 5 minutes.

Keto Egg, Cheese and Bacon Biscuits

Ingredients:

1 cup almond flour

4 egg whites

1/3 cup grass-fed butter

1 t baking powder

1/2 t salt

4 pieces of speck, prosciutto, pancetta, bacon or sausage patties, cooked crispy

4 eggs, fried

4 slices raw, grass-fed sharp cheddar cheese

4 tablespoon of your favorite jam

Instructions:

Biscuits

In a mixer (or with a fork) add together the butter and almond flour and mix until you have small broken up bits of butter. Add the egg whites, salt, and baking powder and mix well. On a greased or lined baking sheet, scoop the batter into 4 even portions. Bake at 350F for about 20 minutes, until slightly golden.

To Assemble

Cut the biscuits in half, spread jam on the top or bottom. Put the egg, then the cheese followed by whichever meat you've crisped up. Place the other half of the biscuit on top and enjoy!

Keto Breakfast Sausage Casserole

Ingredients:

8 eggs, beaten

1 head of chopped cauliflower

1 lb. sausage, cooked and crumbled

2 cups heavy whipping cream

1 cup sharp cheddar cheese, grated

1 teaspoon salt

1 teaspoon dry mustard

Instructions:

Cook sausage.

In a medium bowl add together sausage, heavy whipping cream, chopped cauliflower, cheese, eggs, salt and mustard and mix well.

Pour into a 9×13 casserole dish that has been sprayed with Non-stick spray.

Cook for 45 minutes at 350F or until firm.

Remove and top with more cheese.

Cheesy Buffalo Scrambled Mug Eggs

Ingredients:

Coffee Mug

2 eggs

Salt and pepper

Shredded cheese

Your favorite buffalo wing sauce

Instructions:

Crack eggs into a coffee mug, whisk eggs with fork.

Put the mug into your microwave and cook for 1.5 – 2 minutes, depending on the power of your microwave.

Remove the mug from the microwave (careful, may be hot).

Sprinkle with salt and pepper.

Then, add on your desired amount of cheese.

Using a fork, mix everything together.

Add your buffalo or hot sauce and mix again.

Serve and enjoy!

Breakfast Keto Hash

Ingredients:

1 medium zucchini (6.9 oz)

2 slices bacon

½ small white onion or 1 clove garlic

1 tablespoon ghee or coconut oil

1 tablespoon freshly chopped parsley or chives

¼ teaspoon salt

1 large egg, free-range or organic on top

½ avocado

Instructions:

Finely chop the onion (or garlic) and cut the bacon.

Cook the onion over medium heat and add the bacon, cook until lightly browned.

Meanwhile, dice the zucchini into medium pieces.

Add the zucchini to the pan and cook for 10-15 minutes.

Remove and add chopped parsley.

Serve and Enjoy!

Keto Breakfast Banana Chia Seed Pudding

Ingredients:

1 Can Coconut Milk (full fat)

1 Medium or small size banana, ripe

1/2 teaspoon Cinnamon

1/2 teaspoon Salt

1 teaspoon Vanilla Extract

1/4 cup Chia Seeds

Instructions:

In a medium size bowl mash the banana until soft.

Combine the rest of the ingredients and mix until combined.

Cover and place in the refrigerator overnight (or at least 2 hours).

Enjoy when ready!

Chapter 9:
Main Meal Recipes

Joseph's Keto Pita Pizza

Ingredients:

1 Joseph's Low Carb Pita

½ Cup Rao's Homemade Tomato Basil Marinara Sauce

2 Oz Cheddar Cheese

1 Oz Roasted Red Peppers

14 slices Pepperoni

Instructions:

Place half of the Low Carb Pita on a foil lined sheet.

Rub with some olive oil and crisp it by toasting for 1-2 minutes at 450F.

Spread the sauce over the Pita bread then cover with cheese and toppings.

Cook for another five minutes to melt the cheese, then serve while hot.

Roasted Brussels Sprouts and Prosciutto Bites

Ingredients:

1 pound small Brussels sprouts, rinsed of any dirt

2 tablespoons extra-virgin olive oil

1/4 pound thinly sliced prosciutto

1 pinch coarse salt and freshly ground pepper

Instructions:

Preheat the oven to 400°F.

Slice the Brussels sprouts into halves, lengthwise (do not trim the ends as they will hold together better with them). Toss the sprouts on a rimmed baking sheet with oil and sprinkle with salt and pepper.

Bake for up to 40 minutes, but begin checking at around the 25 minute mark. Feel free to toss them around a bit too.

Chop the prosciutto into small chunks. Heat a medium-sized skillet over medium to high heat. Add the prosciutto and sauté for about 5 minutes, or until nice and crispy, then set aside.

Remove the sprouts from the oven and allow them to cool for about 5 minutes, or until you can handle them.

Use a toothpick to slide on a couple of sprout halves, followed by a slice or 3 of the ham, then bookend it with another sprout half. Continue this way until you have about 32 mini skewers. Arrange on a platter and serve immediately.

Keto Broccoli Cheese Pie

Ingredients:

1 average broccoli (8.8 oz.)

1 cup grated parmesan cheese (2.1 oz.)

3 large eggs (free range or organic)

4 tbsp. fresh full-fat cream

6 anchovies

2 tbsp. extra virgin olive oil

salt and pepper to taste

½ cup micro greens for garnish

Instructions:

Preheat the oven to 300F.

Cut the washed broccoli into florets.

Transfer them into a steamer for about 5-8 minutes or until the stalks are slightly tender.

When done, transfer them into a bowl and blend until smooth.

Add grated parmesan cheese, eggs and cream then mix well as you season with salt and pepper.

Spoon the mixture into silicone forms equally.

Note: Silicone forms are the best I tried for the recipe: nothing gets stuck on them and you can easily empty them. It is advisable to bake them in a water bath as this prevents the top part from drying and cracking.

Place the silicone forms on a baking tray and add 2 cm or 1 inch of water into the tray.

Place in the oven and bake it for 40 minutes.

When this is done, set aside and let them cool.

Finely chop the anchovies and mix them with olive oil.

Remove the cakes from the forms once they are chilled, spoon anchovies on the top and garnish with micro greens.

Enjoy your meal now!

Easy Keto Skirt Steak Fajitas

Ingredients:

Filling

1 small Onion

1 medium Bell Pepper

3 medium Jalapenos

1 small Red Chili Pepper

2 lbs. Skirt Steak

2 teaspoon Cumin

1/2 can Whole Tomatoes

1 tablespoon Apple Cider Vinegar

3 tablespoon Ketchup

1 teaspoon Liquid Smoke

1 teaspoon Minced Garlic

Salt & Pepper

Tortillas

1/4 cup Coconut Flour

1 tablespoon Ground Psyllium Husk

2 tablespoon Butter

1/2 cup Chicken or Beef Broth

1 pinch Garlic Powder

1 pinch Seasoning Salt

Instructions:

Remove silver skin from skirt steak if your butcher missed any.

Cut up all vegetables into bite-size pieces.

Remove seeds from jalapenos and red chili if you don't like much spice.

Combine all ingredients to the crock pot

Cook on low for 6-8 hours.

When you're ready, make your tortillas by boiling the broth and then mixing it into the other ingredients.

Form a dough and cut small circles out.

Fry each circle in a pan on the stove (medium-low heat) until they have browned.

Add fillings of your choice. Enjoy!

Keto Turkey Meatballs

Ingredients:

10 slices Bacon

2 lbs. Ground Turkey

3 small Red Chilies

1/2 medium Green Pepper

1 small Onion

1/2 teaspoon Salt

1/2 teaspoon Pepper

2 large handfuls of spinach

3 sprigs Thyme

2 large Eggs

1 oz. Pork Rinds

Instructions:

Preheat the oven to 400F.

Line a baking sheet with foil and add your bacon.

Cook for 30 minutes or until crisp.

Meanwhile, prep all ingredients by adding to food processor and dicing.

Add all ingredients (except bacon) to the ground turkey and mix well.

Once bacon is cooked, set bacon aside and drain fat into separate container.

Make 20 meatballs and lay over the same sheet the bacon cooked on.

Cook meatballs for 15-20 minutes or until juices run clear, then skewer 2-3 pieces of bacon to each meatball.

In the food processor, combine spinach, bacon fat, and seasonings of your choosing, create "stick" of butter and serve under meatballs.

Enjoy!

Keto Bacon & Chicken Patties

Ingredients:

1 12 Oz Can Chicken Breast

4 Slices Bacon

2 Medium Bell Peppers

1/4 Cup Sun Dried Tomato Pesto

1/4 Cup Parmesan Cheese

1 Large Egg

3 Tablespoon Coconut Flour

Instructions:

Cook bacon until crispy.

In a food processor, finely chop 2 bell peppers and then scoop mixture into a bowl. Remove any excess moisture out with paper towels.

Chop chicken and bacon together in food processor until almost smooth. Add to pepper mixture.

Add parmesan, egg, coconut flour and tomato pesto into the mixture and mix everything together. Make patties with hand and fry on medium heat in a pan with some oil. Once browned, flip over, continue cooking, and remove to paper towels when finished. Enjoy!

Keto Chicken Satay

Ingredients:

1 lb. Ground Chicken

4 Tablespoon Soy Sauce

3 Tablespoon Peanut Butter

2 Spring Onions

1/3 Yellow Pepper

1 Tablespoon Erythritol

1 Tablespoon Rice Vinegar

2 teaspoon Sesame Oil

2 teaspoon Chili Paste

1 teaspoon Minced Garlic

1/4 teaspoon Cayenne

1/4 teaspoon Paprika

Juice of 1/2 Lime

Instructions:

Heat 2 teaspoons sesame oil on medium-high heat in a pan. Add chicken to the pan and cook until brown. Once chicken is cooked, add all other ingredients. Stir well and continue cooking.

Once everything is cooked, add 2 chopped spring onions and 1/3 sliced yellow pepper for garnish.

Keto Low Carb Cumin Crusted Pork Chops

Ingredients:

Crust

1 1/2 lb. Pork Chops

1/4 Cup Golden Flaxseed

3 Tablespoon Coconut Oil (For Frying)

2 teaspoon Cumin

1 teaspoon Coriander

1 teaspoon Cardamom

Salt, Pepper

Vegetables

1 Orange Pepper

1/2 Onion

2 Stalks Celery

1/4 Cup White Wine

Salt, Pepper

Instructions:

Season outside of pork chops with salt and pepper.

Add together all crust ingredients.

Dip pork chops into the flax and spices, fully covering pork chops.

In a cast iron skillet, bring 3 Tablespoon of coconut oil to temperature, add pork chops to pan.

Let them crisp on one side, then flip and reduce heat to medium-low.

Continue cooking until internal temperature of 145F.

Take off pork chops from pan and rest in foil.

With remaining pan juices, add all vegetables and season with salt and pepper.

Add White Wine and cook vegetables until soft.

Serve with extra juices.

Keto Cauliflower and Curry Shrimp

Ingredients:

24 Oz. Shrimp

5 Cups Raw Spinach

4 Cups Chicken Stock

1 Medium Onion

1 teaspoon Onion powder

1 teaspoon Cayenne

1 teaspoon Paprika

1/2 teaspoon Ginger (ground, dried)

1/2 teaspoon Coriander

1/2 teaspoon Turmeric

1/2 teaspoon Pepper

1/4 teaspoon Cardamom

1/4 teaspoon Cinnamon

1/4 teaspoon Xanthan Gum

Salt + Pepper to taste

1/2 Head Medium Cauliflower

1 Cup Unsweetened Coconut Milk

1/4 Cup Butter

1/4 Cup Heavy Cream

3 Tablespoon Olive Oil

2 Tablespoon Curry Powder

1 Tablespoon Coconut Flour

1 Tablespoon Cumin

2 teaspoon Garlic Powder

1 teaspoon Chili Powder

Instructions:

Stir all spices together (except xanthan and coconut flour) set aside.

Slice 1 medium onion into slices. Bring 3 tablespoon olive oil to hot heat in a pan. Add onion, cook onion till soft. Add butter, heavy cream 1/8 teaspoon xanthan and spices, mix well.

After about 1-2 mins of the spices sweating, add 4 cups chicken broth, and 1 cup coconut milk. Mix well, cover and cook for 30 minutes.

Meanwhile, chop cauliflower into small florets then add to curry. Cook for another 15 minutes, covered.

Add shrimp to the curry. Cook for an additional 10-20 minutes with the lid off.

Add coconut flour and 1/8 teaspoon xanthan gum and mix well into curry. Let cook for 5 minutes.

After 5 minutes, add spinach and mix it in well. Cook for an addition 5-10 minutes with the lid off. Enjoy!

Keto Bacon & Chicken Sausage Stir Fry

Ingredients:

4 Cheddar & Bacon Chicken Sausages

3 Cups Broccoli Florets

3 Cups Spinach

1/2 Cup Parmesan Cheese

1/2 Cup Rao's Tomato Sauce

1/4 Cup Red Wine (Merlot)

2 Tablespoon Salted Butter

2 teaspoon Minced Garlic

1/2 teaspoon Pepper

1/2 teaspoon Red Pepper Flakes

1/2 teaspoon Kosher Salt

Instructions:

Cut the sausages into slices.

Start to boil water on the stove.

Meanwhile, add your sausage to a pan on high heat.

Add your broccoli to the boiling water and cook for 3-5 minutes.

Cook your sausages until they brown on both sides.

Transfer your sausages to one side of the pan, then add the butter.

Put your garlic in the butter and let it cook for 1 minute.

Add everything together and then add your broccoli.

Pour in the tomato sauce, red wine, and add red pepper flakes.

Stir together, add your spinach with salt and pepper and let it cool down.

Simmer this for 5-10 minutes.

Enjoy!

Keto Fiery Buffalo Strips

Ingredients:

5 Chicken Breasts Pounded to 1/2" Thickness

3/4 Cup Almond Flour

1/2 Cup Hot Sauce

1/4 Cup Olive Oil

3 Tablespoon Butter

3 Tablespoon Blue Cheese Crumbles

2 Large Eggs

1 Tablespoon Paprika

1 Tablespoon Chili powder

2 teaspoon Salt

2 teaspoon Pepper

1 teaspoon Garlic Powder

1 teaspoon Onion Powder

Instructions:

Preheat oven to 400F.

In a ramekin, combine paprika, chili powder, salt, pepper, garlic powder, and onion powder.

Pound out chicken breasts to 1/2" thickness, then cut the chicken breasts in half.

Spread 1/3 of the spice mix over the chicken breast, then flip them over and do the same with 1/3 of the spice mix.

In a bowl, add together almond flour and 1/3 of the spice mix. In another container, crack 2 eggs and whisk them.

Dip each piece of seasoned chicken into the spice mix and then into the almond flour, coating well.

Place each piece on a cooling rack on top of a foiled baking sheet.

Cook the chicken for 15 minutes.

Take the chicken out of the oven and turn your oven to broil.

Drizzle 2 Tablespoon Olive Oil over the chicken.

Broil for 5 minutes, flip the breasts, drizzle with remaining olive oil, and broil again for 5 minutes.

In a sauce pan, combined 1/2 Cup of hot sauce with 3 Tablespoon Butter.

Serve chicken with slathering of hot sauce and blue cheese crumbles.

Keto Roasted Rosemary Chicken Thighs

Ingredients:

7 Skinless, Boneless Chicken Thigh

1 Tablespoon Minced Garlic

3 Tablespoon Olive Oil

2 Large Lemons

2 Tablespoon Fresh Thyme

3 teaspoon Kosher Salt

1 1/2 teaspoon Dried Rosemary

1 1/2 teaspoon Dried Ground Sage

1/2 teaspoon Ground Black Pepper

Instructions:

In a mortar, add garlic and 2 teaspoons kosher salt.

Grind the garlic and salt together with a pestle, creating a paste.

Slowly add your oil, grinding and mixing into a paste.

Once the paste is ready, dry your chicken off and put it into a bag with the paste.

Coat the chicken well.

Marinate the chicken for anywhere from 2-10 hours.

Preheat your oven to 425F.

Slice 2 lemons thin and arrange the slices on the bottom of a baking pan.

Lay your chicken on top of the lemons.

Remove the thyme leaves from the stem and add your thyme, rosemary, sage, pepper, and remaining salt to the chicken.

Bake for 25-30 minutes, or until the juices run clear.

Chapter 10: Dessert Recipes

Chocolate Coconut Candies

Ingredients:

1 cup extra virgin coconut oil (7 oz.)

1 cup raw cocoa powder (3.5 oz.)

1 tsp. pure vanilla bean extract (1-2 vanilla beans)

¼ cup Erythritol, powdered or other healthy low-carb sweetener from this list

10-15 drops Stevia extract (Clear / Coconut)

A pinch of salt

¼ cup homemade coconut & pecan butter, chilled (1.7 oz.)

Instructions:

Place the extra virgin coconut oil in a small bowl and melt it in a microwave oven on low heat for about 1 minute.

Add raw cocoa powder, vanilla extract, stevia and Erythritol (Note that Erythritol doesn't dissolve easily unless heated up, you can also blend it to obtain a smoother texture).

Mix everything well, ensuring there are no clumps.

Spoon the chocolate mixture into the silicone about 1/3 of the way full.

Refrigerate the molds for about 15-30 minutes, or until the chocolate mixture solidifies.

Add ½ a teaspoon of homemade coconut and pecan butter into the mold (the best results are achieved when the butter is chilled).

Top with the remaining chocolate mixture and return to the fridge for another 30-60 minutes or until firm.

Once this is done, keep the molds refrigerated since coconut oil gets very soft at room temperature.

Keto Cherry Danish

Ingredients:

Pastry

3 extra large eggs, separated (reserving ½ of the yolks for filling)

¼ teaspoon cream of tartar

¼ cup Swerve (or 1 tsp. stevia glycerite)

1 teaspoon cherry extract

3 Tablespoon sour cream (or coconut cream if dairy free)

¼ cup Jay Robb Strawberry OR Vanilla Egg White Protein or Whey Protein

Filling

4 oz. cream cheese, softened (or coconut cream if dairy allergy)

½ of the egg yolks from above

¼ cup Swerve (or ½ tsp. stevia glycerite)

1 tsp. cherry extract (or other like lemon/strawberry/blueberry/almond/raspberry)

Drizzle

1 oz. cream cheese, softened

1 TBS Swerve confectioners (or a drop of stevia glycerite)

¼ tsp. cherry extract (or other extract)

Instructions:

Pastry Directions

Separate the egg white from the yolks, putting the egg white in a large bowl and the yolks in a relatively smaller bowl. Put half of the yolk in a little dish, reserve this for filling. Use an electric beater to whip the egg white and tartar cream until very stiff, then add protein powder.

To the other half of yolks, add sour cream and natural sweetener and beat well until smooth.

Using a big spatula, fold the yolk mixture into the egg whites gently, being careful to get it well blended. Grease a cookie sheet and plop 6 equal mounds of mixture to make 6 Danishes. Make an indent on each mound and fill with filling.

Filling directions

Soften cream cheese and add the remaining half of egg yolks, sweeteners, extract and flavoring. Fill the pastries and bake for about 20-30 minutes at 300F or until golden brown. Remove and allow to cool.

Directions to make the drizzle

Warm the cream cheese and stir in the natural sweetener and extract. Place the resulting mixture in a piping bag (or let it cool and use a small zip lock and cut a tiny hole into the corner) then drizzle over the cooled Danish.

Decadent Baked Keto Strawberry Cheesecake

Ingredients:

Crust

¾ Cup Pecans (84g)

¾ Cup Almond Flour

4 Tbsp. Butter

2 Tbsp. Splenda

Filling

1½ lbs. Cream Cheese

4 Eggs

½ Tbsp. Liquid Vanilla

½ Tbsp. Lemon Juice

½ tsp. EZ-Sweetz (Equivalent to 1 cup sugar, if Splenda, use 1 cup)

¼ Cup Sour Cream

9 Strawberries

Instructions:

Crust

Preheat to oven to 400 degrees.

Crush the pecans.

In a saucepan, melt butter and add pecans, Splenda and flour and mix for several minutes.

Grease a 9" spring form pan and add the dough.

Cook for 7 minutes until it starts to brown.

Filling

Combine all ingredients at room temperature.

Mix well.

Slice and Place strawberries along the sides of the crust and fill with filling.

Place in oven and lower heat to 250 degrees.

Bake 60-90 minutes.

Creamy Chocoberry Fudge Sauce

Ingredients:

4 ounces cream cheese, softened

1-3.5 ounce bar Lindt 90% chocolate, chopped

1/4 cup powdered erythritol

1/4 cup of heavy cream

2 tbsp. Monin sugar free Raspberry Syrup

Instructions:

Melt together cream cheese and chocolate.

Once melted, stir in sweetener.

Remove from heat and let cool.

Once cool, mix in cream and syrup.

Mix well and serve over fruit or homemade ice cream.

Easy Choco-Coconut Pudding

Ingredients:

1 cup coconut milk (full fat, canned)

2 tbsp. cacao powder or organic cocoa

1/2 tsp. stevia powder extract

Or 2 Tbsp. honey or maple syrup

1 Tbsp. quality gelatin

2 Tbsp. water

Instructions:

Over medium heat whisk together coconut milk, cocoa, and sweetener.

In a separate bowl, mix the gelatin and water.

Add to pan and stir until fully dissolved.

Pour into small dishes and refrigerate 30-45 minutes until set.

Exotic Cupcakes

Ingredients:

Cupcakes

1/2 cup coconut flour

1/2 cup granulated erythritol

1/4 cup unsweetened cocoa

(optional)

1/4 teaspoon baking soda

1/4 teaspoon sea salt

6 eggs

1/2 cup coconut oil, OR butter melted

1 tablespoon vanilla extract

1 teaspoon Stevia glycerite

Filling

1 cup heavy cream

1 teaspoon Stevia glycerite, OR to taste

Frosting

8 oz. cream cheese, softened

1/4 cup unsweetened vanilla almond milk

1 teaspoon Stevia glycerite

Chocolate Stripes

3 tablespoon granulated erythritol

2 oz. unsweetened chocolate, chopped

3 tablespoon unsweetened vanilla almond milk

1 teaspoon vanilla extract

1/4 teaspoon Stevia glycerite

Instructions:

Preheat oven to 350 degrees.

Sift together coconut flour, erythritol, cocoa, baking soda and salt.

In a separate bowl, beat eggs. Stir in coconut oil/butter, vanilla extract and Stevia.

Slowly incorporate the wet ingredients into the dry ingredients. Mix until smooth. Pour into greased muffin tins 1/3 full. Bake 13-18 minutes.

Once cool, cut cupcakes in half. Whip the cream and add the Stevia. Fill middle of cupcake with 2 tbsp. whipped cream. Put cupcakes back together and freeze for 2 hours.

Mix together cream cheese, vanilla almond milk and Stevia. Dip frozen cupcakes in icing.

Grind granulated erythritol into a powder. Melt together chocolate and almond milk. Mix in the erythritol, vanilla extract and Stevia until smooth.

Drizzle over cupcakes and try not to eat them all at once!

Microwave Tiramisu

Ingredients:

Cake Mixture

1 tbsp. erythritol or any sweetener of choice

1/2 tsp. of LC sweet brown sugar without the carbs, you can omit this if you want

1 tbsp. of unsalted soften butter

3 tbsp. of almond flour (Honeyville brand)

2 tbsp. of vanilla whey protein powder

1/4 tsp. of baking powder

1 tbsp. of almond milk

2 tbsp. of beaten egg or egg whites

Coffee Mixture

1 tbsp. of instant coffee

2 tbsp. of water

Filling

2 oz. cream cheese (or if you have mascarpone cheese, use that)

2 tbsp. whipped cream or heavy cream

1 tsp. of erythritol

Garnish

1 tsp. unsweetened cocoa powder

1 tsp. of unsweetened grated chocolate

Instructions:

Cake Mixture

First, mix together the sweetener and the softened butter.

Next, mix in the rest of the ingredients.

Divide into 2 ramekins.

Wait 1 minute for baking powder to activate.

Microwave for 1 minute.

Filling

Melt cream cheese in microwave for 30 seconds and mix in cream and sweetener.

To Assemble

Cut cake in half.

Dip 2 pieces of cake into coffee mixture.

Layer the cake with the filling and sprinkle with cocoa and grated chocolate.

Conclusion

Thank you again for downloading this book!

I do hope that you have found that this is an easy introduction to the Ketogenic way of eating and I hope that you are inspired to make a change in your life starting today.

All that is left is for you to get started and here I urge you, don't wait too long - this is not something that should be put off until after the weekend or until Monday! Start today if you can - at the very least, clear out the banned food from your grocery cupboard.

I wish you the very best going forward. I sincerely hope that you derive as much benefit from the ketogenic lifestyle as I have.

Finally, I would really appreciate if you could review this book for me and update me on your progress on Amazon - I would love to hear from you! If you really enjoyed this book, keep your eyes open for my upcoming Super Foods Series available exclusively in the Amazon bookstore.

Best wishes for the new, healthier you.

Thank you and good luck!

Made in the USA
Lexington, KY
30 May 2016